Medical Ethics

Physicians and Patients

Akmal El-Mazny

CONTENTS

INTRODUCTION

"Ethics consists of knowing what is right to do and what is wrong to avoid" (Socrates; 470-399 BC).

Medical ethics refers to a system of moral principles that apply values and judgments to medical practice.

Ethics is and always has been an essential component of physician-patient relationship, which facilitates the exchange of medical knowledge and care within a framework of trust.

The basic principles of medical ethics include: autonomy (respect of the patient preferences), beneficence (taking actions that serve the best interests of patients), non-maleficence (first, do no harm), and justice (fairness and equality).

This book is structured to address issues related to medical ethics in which physicians are involved, but at the core will always be the relationship between physicians and patients.

I hope this book will reinforce and strengthen your ethical mindset and provide tools to deal with the ethical issues that you will encounter in your medical practice.

ETHICS THEORIES

Dealing with moral issues is often perplexing:

– How, exactly, should we think through an ethical issue?

– What questions should we ask?

– What factors should we consider?

Philosophers have developed five different theories for approaches to deal with moral issues:

Virtue Approach Theory

"Virtue is the way we act to gain our values" (Socrates; 470-399 BC).

The virtue approach to ethics assumes that there are certain ideals toward which we should strive, which provide for the full development of our humanity.

These ideals are discovered through thoughtful reflection on what kind of people we have the potential to become.

Virtues are attitudes or character traits that enable us to be and to act in ways that develop our highest potential.

They enable us to pursue the ideals we have adopted; honesty, courage, compassion, generosity, fidelity, integrity, fairness, self-control, and prudence are all examples of virtues.

Virtues are like habits; that are, once acquired; they become characteristic of a person.

Moreover, a person who has developed virtues will be naturally disposed to act in ways consistent with moral principles; the virtuous person is the ethical person.

In dealing with an ethical problem using the virtue approach, we might ask:

– What kind of person should I be?

– What will promote the development of character within myself and my community?

Fairness or Justice Approach Theory

The fairness or justice approach to ethics has its roots in the teachings of the ancient Greek philosopher Aristotle (384-322 BC), who said that "equals should be treated equally and unequals unequally".

The basic moral question in this approach is:

– How fair is an action?

– Does it treat everyone in the same way?

– Does it show favoritism and discrimination?

Favoritism gives benefits to some people without a justifiable reason for singling them out.

Discrimination imposes burdens on people who are no different from those on whom burdens are not imposed.

Both favoritism and discrimination are unjust and wrong.

Rights Approach Theory

The rights approach to ethics has its roots in the philosophy of the 18th century thinker Immanuel Kant and others like him, who focused on the individual's right to choose for himself.

According to these philosophers, what makes human beings different from mere things is that people have dignity based on their ability to choose freely what they will do with their lives, and they have a fundamental moral right to have these choices respected.

People are not objects to be manipulated; it is a violation of human dignity to use people in ways they do not freely choose.

Of course, many different, but related, rights exist besides this basic one:

– The right to the truth: We have a right to be told the truth and to be informed about matters that significantly affect our choices.

– The right of privacy: We have the right to do, believe, and say whatever we choose in our personal lives so long as we do not violate the rights of others.

– The right not to be injured: We have the right not to be harmed or injured unless we freely and knowingly do something to deserve punishment or we freely and knowingly choose to risk such injuries.

– The right to what is agreed: We have a right to what has been promised by those with whom we have freely entered into agreement.

In deciding whether an action is moral or immoral using this approach, then, we must ask: Does the action respect the moral rights of everyone?

Utilitarian Approach Theory

Utilitarianism was conceived in the 19th century by Jeremy Bentham and John Stuart Mill to help legislators determine which laws were morally best.

Both Bentham and Mill suggested that ethical actions are those that provide the greatest balance of good over evil.

To analyze an issue using the utilitarian approach:

− First identify the various courses of action available to us.

− Second, we ask who will be affected by each action and what benefits or harms will be derived from each.

− Third, we choose the action that will produce the greatest benefits and the least harm.

The ethical action is the one that provides the greatest good for the greatest number.

Common-Good Approach Theory

This approach to ethics assumes a society comprising individuals whose own good is inextricably linked to the good of the community.

Community members are bound by the pursuit of common values and goals.

The common good is a notion that originated more than 2,000 years ago in the writings of Plato, Aristotle, and Cicero.

More recently, contemporary ethicist John Rawls defined the common good as "certain general conditions that are equally to everyone's advantage".

In this approach, we focus on ensuring that the social policies, social systems, institutions, and environments on which we depend are beneficial to all.

Examples of goods common to all include affordable health care, effective public safety, peace among nations, a just legal system, and an unpolluted environment.

Appeals to the common good urge us to view ourselves as members of the same community, reflecting on broad questions concerning the kind of society we want to become and how we are to achieve that society.

While respecting and valuing the freedom of individuals to pursue their own goals, the common-good approach challenges us also to recognize and further those goals we share in common.

HUMAN RIGHTS

The human rights era started with the formation of the United Nations in 1945, which was charged with the promotion of human rights.

The Universal Declaration of Human Rights (1948) was the first major document to define human rights.

Article 1

All human beings are born free and equal in dignity and rights.

They are endowed with reason and conscience and should act towards one another in a spirit of brotherhood.

Article 2

Everyone is entitled to all the rights and freedoms set forth in this Declaration, without distinction of any kind, such as race, colour, sex, language, religion, political or other opinion, national or social origin, property, birth or other status.

Furthermore, no distinction shall be made on the basis of the political, jurisdictional or international status of the country or territory to which a person belongs, whether it be independent, trust, non-self-governing or under any other limitation of sovereignty.

Article 3

Everyone has the right to life, liberty and security of person.

Article 4

No one shall be held in slavery or servitude; slavery and the slave trade shall be prohibited in all their forms.

Article 5

No one shall be subjected to torture or to cruel, inhuman or degrading treatment or punishment.

Article 6

Everyone has the right to recognition everywhere as a person before the law.

Article 7

All are equal before the law and are entitled without any discrimination to equal protection of the law.

All are entitled to equal protection against any discrimination in violation of this Declaration and against any incitement to such discrimination.

Article 8

Everyone has the right to an effective remedy by the competent national tribunals for acts violating the fundamental rights granted him by the constitution or by law.

Article 9

No one shall be subjected to arbitrary arrest, detention or exile.

Article 10

Everyone is entitled in full equality to a fair and public hearing by an independent and impartial tribunal, in the determination of his rights and obligations and of any criminal charge against him.

Article 11

1. Everyone charged with a penal offence has the right to be presumed innocent until proved guilty according to law in a public trial at which he has had all the guarantees necessary for his defence.

2. No one shall be held guilty of any penal offence on account of any act or omission which did not constitute a penal offence, under national or international law, at the time when it was committed.

   Nor shall a heavier penalty be imposed than the one that was applicable at the time the penal offence was committed.

Article 12

No one shall be subjected to arbitrary interference with his privacy, family, home or correspondence, nor to attacks upon his honour and reputation.

Everyone has the right to the protection of the law against such interference or attacks.

Article 13

1. Everyone has the right to freedom of movement and residence within the borders of each State.

2. Everyone has the right to leave any country, including his own, and to return to his country.

Article 14

1. Everyone has the right to seek and to enjoy in other countries asylum from persecution.

2. This right may not be invoked in the case of prosecutions genuinely arising from non-political crimes or from acts contrary to the purposes and principles of the United Nations.

Article 15

1. Everyone has the right to a nationality.

2. No one shall be arbitrarily deprived of his nationality nor denied the right to change his nationality.

Article 16

1. Men and women of full age, without any limitation due to race, nationality or religion, have the right to marry and to found a family.

   They are entitled to equal rights as to marriage, during marriage and at its dissolution.

2. Marriage shall be entered into only with the free and full consent of the intending spouses.

3. The family is the natural and fundamental group unit of society and is entitled to protection by society and the State.

Article 17

1. Everyone has the right to own property alone as well as in association with others.

2. No one shall be arbitrarily deprived of his property.

Article 18

Everyone has the right to freedom of thought, conscience and religion; including freedom to change his religion or belief, and freedom, either alone or in community with others and in public or private, to manifest his religion or belief in teaching, practice, worship and observance.

Article 19

Everyone has the right to freedom of opinion and expression; this right includes freedom to hold opinions without interference and to seek, receive and impart information and ideas through any media and regardless of frontiers.

Article 20

1. Everyone has the right to freedom of peaceful assembly and association.

2. No one may be compelled to belong to an association.

Article 21

1. Everyone has the right to take part in the government of his country, directly or through freely chosen representatives.

2. Everyone has the right to equal access to public service in his country.

3. The will of the people shall be the basis of the authority of government; this will shall be expressed in periodic and genuine elections which shall be by universal and equal suffrage and shall be held by secret vote or by equivalent free voting procedures.

Article 22

Everyone, as a member of society, has the right to social security and is entitled to realization, through national effort and international co-operation and in accordance with the organization and resources of each State, of the economic, social and cultural rights indispensable for his dignity and the free development of his personality.

Article 23

1. Everyone has the right to work, to free choice of employment, to just and favourable conditions of work and to protection against unemployment.

2. Everyone, without any discrimination, has the right to equal pay for equal work.

3. Everyone who works has the right to just and favourable remuneration ensuring for himself and his family an existence worthy of human dignity, and supplemented, if necessary, by other means of social protection.

4. Everyone has the right to form and to join trade unions for the protection of his interests.

Article 24

Everyone has the right to rest and leisure, including reasonable limitation of working hours and periodic holidays with pay.

Article 25

1. Everyone has the right to a standard of living adequate for the health and well-being of himself and of his family, including food, clothing, housing and medical care and necessary social services, and the right to security in the event of unemployment, sickness, disability, widowhood, old age or other lack of livelihood in circumstances beyond his control.

2. Motherhood and childhood are entitled to special care and assistance.

   All children, whether born in or out of wedlock, shall enjoy the same social protection.

Article 26

1. Everyone has the right to education.

   Education shall be free, at least in the elementary and fundamental stages.

   Elementary education shall be compulsory.

   Technical and professional education shall be made generally available and higher education shall be equally accessible to all on the basis of merit.

2. Education shall be directed to the full development of the human personality and to the strengthening of respect for human rights and fundamental freedoms.

   It shall promote understanding, tolerance and friendship among all nations, racial or religious groups, and shall further the activities of the UN for the maintenance of peace.

3. Parents have a prior right to choose the kind of education that shall be given to their children.

Article 27

1. Everyone has the right freely to participate in the cultural life of the community, to enjoy the arts and to share in scientific advancement and its benefits.

2. Everyone has the right to the protection of the moral and material interests resulting from any scientific, literary or artistic production of which he is the author.

Article 28

Everyone is entitled to a social and international order in which the rights and freedoms set forth in this Declaration can be fully realized.

Article 29

1. Everyone has duties to the community in which alone the free and full development of his personality is possible.

2. In the exercise of his rights and freedoms, everyone shall be subject only to such limitations as are determined by law solely for the purpose of securing due recognition and respect for the rights and freedoms of others and of meeting the just requirements of morality, public order and the general welfare in a democratic society.

3. These rights and freedoms may in no case be exercised contrary to the purposes and principles of the United Nations.

Article 30

Nothing in this Declaration may be interpreted as implying for any State, group or person any right to engage in any activity or to perform any act aimed at the destruction of any of the rights and freedoms set forth herein.

ETHICS AND MEDICINE

Medicine is both a science and an art.

Science deals with what can be observed and measured, and a competent physician recognizes the signs of illness and disease and knows how to restore good health.

But scientific medicine has its limits, particularly in regard to human individuality, culture, religion, freedom, rights and responsibilities.

The art of medicine involves the application of medical science and technology to individual patients, families and communities, no two of which are identical.

By far the major part of the differences among individuals, families and communities is non-physiological, and it is in recognizing and dealing with these differences that the arts, humanities and social sciences, along with ethics, play a major role.

Actually all the ethical theories are applied in medical practice:

−Character: Virtue ethics (Plato, Aristotle).

−Doing right: Duties and respect of others (Kant).

−Social responsibility: Justice (Aristotle) and utilitarianism (Benthan and Mill).

HISTORY OF MEDICAL ETHICS

Historically, Western medical ethics may be traced to guidelines on the duty of physicians in antiquity, such as the Hippocratic Oath (400 BC).

It has addressed two main areas:

– The ethical attitude towards other physicians.

– The clinical practice dealing with a physician's duty to his patients.

However, the oath did not consider the patient's right of choice in the management of his medical problem.

The first code of medical ethics, "Formula Comitis Archiatrorum", was published in the 5th century; during the reign of the Ostrogothic king Theodoric the Great.

In the medieval and early modern period, the field is indebted to:

– Islamic scholarship such as Ishaq ibn Ali al-Ruhawi (who wrote the Conduct of a Physician, the first book dedicated to medical ethics), Avicenna's Canon of Medicine and Muhammad ibn Zakariya ar-Razi (known as Rhazes in the West).

– Roman Catholic scholastic thinkers such as Thomas Aquinas, and the case-oriented analysis (casuistry) of Catholic moral theology.

– Jewish thinkers such as Maimonides.

These intellectual traditions continue in Islamic, Catholic, and Jewish medical ethics.

By the 18th and 19th centuries, medical ethics emerged as a more self-conscious discourse.

In England, Thomas Percival, a physician and author, crafted the first modern code of medical ethics.

He drew up a pamphlet with the code in 1794 and wrote an expanded version in 1803, in which he coined the expressions "medical ethics" and "medical jurisprudence".

However, there are some who see Percival's guidelines that relate to physician consultations as being excessively protective of the home physician's reputation.

Jeffrey Berlant is one such critic who considers Percival's codes of physician consultations as being an early example of the anti-competitive, "guild"-like nature of the physician community.

In 1815, the Apothecaries Act was passed by the Parliament of the United Kingdom.

It introduced compulsory apprenticeship and formal qualifications for the apothecaries of the day under the license of the Society of Apothecaries.

This was the beginning of regulation of the medical profession in the UK.

In 1847, the American Medical Association adopted its first code of ethics, with this being based in large part upon Percival's work.

While the secularized field borrowed largely from Catholic medical ethics, in the 20th century a distinctively liberal Protestant approach was articulated by thinkers such as Joseph Fletcher.

The human rights era started with the formation of the United Nations in 1945, which was charged with the promotion of human rights.

The Universal Declaration of Human Rights (1948) was the first major document to define human rights "the equal and inalienable rights of all members of the human family".

The Declaration of Human Rights was followed by several international codes of ethics in medical practice and medical research to protect the patient rights.

The growing influence of ethics in contemporary medicine can be seen in the increasing use of:

– Institutional Review Boards to evaluate experiments on human subjects.

– The establishment of hospital ethics committees.

– The expansion of the role of clinician ethicists.

– The integration of ethics into many medical school curricula.

PRINCIPLES OF MEDICAL ETHICS

A common framework used in the analysis of medical ethics is the "four principles" approach postulated by Tom Beauchamp and James Childress in their textbook "Principles of biomedical ethics".

It recognizes four basic principles, which are to be judged and weighed against each other, with attention given to the scope of their application.

The four basic principles are:

−Autonomy: Respect for the patient's right to refuse or choose their treatment.

−Beneficence: A practitioner should act in the best interest of the patient.

−Non-maleficence: First, do no harm.

−Justice: Concerns the distribution of scarce health resources, and the decision of who gets what treatment (fairness and equality).

Other values that are sometimes discussed include:

−Respect for persons: The patient (and the person treating the patient) has the right to be treated with dignity.

−Truthfulness and honesty: The concept of informed consent has increased in importance since the historical events of the Doctors' Trial of the Nuremberg trials and Tuskegee syphilis experiment.

Values such as these do not give answers as to how to handle a particular situation, but provide a useful framework for understanding conflicts.

When moral values are in conflict, the result may be an ethical dilemma or crisis.

Sometimes, no good solution to a dilemma in medical ethics exists, and, on occasion, the values of the medical community (i.e., the hospital and its staff) conflict with the values of the individual patient, family, or larger non-medical community.

Conflicts can also arise between health care providers, or among family members.

Some argue that the principles of autonomy and beneficence clash, e.g., when patients refuse blood transfusions, considering them life-saving; and truth-telling was not emphasized to a large extent before the HIV era.

AUTONOMY

It is the respect of the patient preferences and treating him as an equal partner in decision-making of all matters related to him.

physicians must provide the patient with all the information that will enable him to make rational and independent decision.

Competent patient (with his own values) should make decisions about diagnosis and treatment.

The patient has the right to:

− Refuse treatment.

− Refuse investigation.

− Give instructions.

− Advanced medical directives: The patient's wishes to be fulfilled in emergency situations or after death.

Paternalism is applied for the incompetent patients:

− Children.

− Unconscious patients.

− Demented patients.

− Mentally retarded patients.

− Emergency situation endangering life.

The principle of autonomy recognizes the rights of individuals to self-determination.

This is rooted in society's respect for individuals' ability to make informed decisions about personal matters.

Autonomy has become more important as social values have shifted to define medical quality in terms of outcomes that are important to the patient rather than medical professionals.

The increasing importance of autonomy can be seen as a social reaction to a "paternalistic" tradition within healthcare.

Some have questioned whether the backlash against historically excessive paternalism in favor of patient autonomy has inhibited the proper use of soft paternalism to the detriment of outcomes for some patients.

Respect for autonomy is the basis for informed consent and advance directives.

Autonomy is a general indicator of health; many diseases are characterised by loss of autonomy, in various manners.

This makes autonomy an indicator for both personal well-being, and for the well-being of the profession.

This has implications for the consideration of medical ethics:

− Is the aim of health care to do good, and benefit from it? Or

− Is the aim of health care to do good to others, and have them, and society, benefit from this?

Ethics - by definition - tries to find a beneficial balance between the activities of the individual and its effects on a collective.

By considering autonomy as a gauge parameter for (self) health care, the medical and ethical perspective both benefit from the implied reference to health.

Psychiatrists and clinical psychologists are often asked to evaluate a patient's capacity for making life-and-death decisions at the end of life.

Persons with a psychiatric condition such as delirium or clinical depression may not have the capacity to make end-of-life decisions.

Therefore, for these persons, a request to refuse treatment may be taken in consideration of their condition and not followed.

Unless there is a clear advance directive to the contrary, in general persons lacking mental capacity are treated according to their best interests.

On the other hand, persons with the mental capacity to make end-of-life decisions have the right to refuse treatment and choose an early death if that is what they truly want.

In such cases, psychiatrists and psychologists are typically part of protecting that right.

BENEFICENCE

The term beneficence refers to actions that promote the well being of others.

In the medical context, this means taking actions that serve the best interests of patients.

Physicians must weigh the risks and benefits when treating their patients, and chose what is most beneficial to them.

However, uncertainty surrounds the precise definition of which practices do in fact help patients.

Tom Beauchamp and James Childress in "Principle of Biomedical Ethics" (1978) identify beneficence as one of the core values of healthcare ethics.

Some scholars, such as Edmund Pellegrino, argue that beneficence is the only fundamental principle of medical ethics.

They argue that healing should be the sole purpose of medicine, and that endeavors like cosmetic surgery and euthanasia fall beyond its purview.

NON-MALEFICENCE

The concept of non-maleficence is embodied by the phrase, "first, do no harm", or the Latin, "primum non nocere".

Many consider that should be the main or primary consideration (hence "primum"): that it is more important not to harm your patient, than to do them good.

All interventions can potentially cause harm, so physicians must chose those where benefits overweigh risks.

This is partly because enthusiastic practitioners are prone to using treatments that they believe will do good, without first having evaluated them adequately to ensure they do no (or only acceptable levels of) harm.

It is not only more important to do no harm than to do good; it is also important to know how likely it is that your treatment will harm a patient.

So a physician should go further than not prescribing medications they know to be harmful - he should not prescribe medications (or otherwise treat the patient) unless he knows that the treatment is unlikely to be harmful; or at the very least, that patient understands the risks and benefits, and that the likely benefits outweigh the likely risks.

In practice, however, many treatments carry some risk of harm.

In some circumstances, e.g., in desperate situations where the outcome without treatment will be grave, risky treatments that stand a high chance of harming the patient will be justified, as the risk of not treating is also very likely to do harm.

So the principle of "non-maleficence" is not absolute, and balances against the principle of "beneficence" (doing good), as the effects of the two principles together often give rise to a "double effect".

Depending on the cultural consensus conditioning (expressed by its religious, political and legal social system) the legal definition of non-maleficence differs.

Violation of non-maleficence is the subject of medical malpractice litigation. Regulations therefore differ over time, per nation.

JUSTICE

Justice is the granting and fulfillment of legitimate rights of others, and injustice is their denial.

Physicians should treat patients equally irrespective to non-medical factors as race, gender, religion, or social standard.

Justice requires the division of rights and assets in an equitable and appropriate manner, but no less so the fair distribution of duties and burdens.

In the simplistic sense, justice means equality.

However, in daily life, many variables cause unequal division of obligations and rights.

Therefore, several ethical theories and techniques have been developed for distributive justice, taking into consideration needs, rights, contributions to society, and other factors.

Different theories of justice place greater priority on different factors: Marxism emphasizes economic needs, while liberalism emphasizes social needs.

The differences in views and emphases make it difficult to attain ideal justice, since equality in one aspect may bring inequality in another and, hence, injustice.

Individual rights became a cornerstone in political, legal and social thinking in the nineteenth century.

Some believe that people have absolute moral rights unrelated to changing social conditions.

These include "natural" universal rights such as the right to life, liberty and privacy.

Others believe that rights flow from societal consensus, customs and laws and therefore are relative and may change according to the circumstances.

RESPECT FOR HUMAN RIGHTS

The human rights era started with the formation of the United Nations in 1945, which was charged with the promotion of human rights.

The Universal Declaration of Human Rights (1948) was the first major document to define human rights.

Physicians have an ethical duty to protect the human rights and human dignity of the patient so the advent of a document that defines human rights has had its effect on medical ethics.

Most codes of medical ethics now require respect for the human rights of the patient.

The Council of Europe promotes the rule of law and observance of human rights in Europe.

The Council of Europe adopted the "European Convention on Human Rights and Biomedicine" (1997) to create a uniform code of medical ethics for its 47 member-states.

The Convention applies international human rights law to medical ethics.

It provides special protection of physical integrity for those who are unable to consent, which includes children.

No organ or tissue removal may be carried out on a person who does not have the capacity to consent under Article 5.

As of December 2013, the Convention had been ratified or acceded to by twenty-nine member-states of the Council of Europe.

The United Nations Educational, Scientific and Cultural Organization (UNESCO) also promotes the protection of human rights and human dignity.

According to UNESCO, Declarations are another means of defining norms, which are not subject to ratification.

Like recommendations, they set forth universal principles to which the community of States wished to attribute the greatest possible authority and to afford the broadest possible support.

UNESCO adopted the "Universal Declaration on Human Rights and Biomedicine" to advance the application of international human rights law in medical ethics.

The Declaration provides special protection of human rights for incompetent persons.

In applying and advancing scientific knowledge, medical practice and associated technologies, human vulnerability should be taken into account.

Individuals and groups of special vulnerability should be protected and the personal integrity of such individuals respected.

COMMUNICATION AND COUNSELLING

Many so-called "ethical conflicts" in medical ethics are traceable back to a lack of communication.

Communication breakdowns between patients and their healthcare team, between family members, or between members of the medical community, can all lead to disagreements and strong feelings.

These breakdowns should be remedied, and many apparently insurmountable "ethics" problems can be solved with communication.

Counselling is the process of assisting and guiding clients, especially by a trained person on a professional basis, to resolve especially, medical, personal, social, or psychological problems and difficulties.

It occurs when a client and counsellor set aside time in order to explore problems and diagnoses which may include the stressful or emotional feelings of the patient.

Counselling helps the patient to see things more clearly, possibly from a different view-point.

This can enable the patient to focus on feelings, experiences or behaviour, with a goal to facilitating positive change towards problems.

Active listening, empathy and body language are paramount to successful counselling.

Counsellor needs to be empathetic, seeing things from the patient's point of view rather than sympathetic (feeling sorry for their patients).

Basic counselling techniques include active listening, body language, asking questions, paraphrasing, and summarizing.

Active listening happens when you "listen for meaning"; the listener says very little but conveys empathy, acceptance and genuiness.

Developing encouraging body language can take some practice; communication is 55% body language, 38% tone and 7% words.

In counselling there is normally a familiar pattern of sessions - introduction, information gathering, discussion, and conclusion.

A summary, in counselling, is when you focus on the main points of a presentation or session in order to highlight them.

Counselling steps include discussion of findings, options, plan, support, and follow-up.

INFORMED CONSENT

Informed consent in ethics usually refers to the idea that a person must be fully informed about and understand the potential benefits and risks of their choice of treatment.

Informed consent is more than simply getting a patient to sign a written consent form; it is a process of communication between a patient and physician that results in the patient's authorization or agreement to undergo a specific medical intervention.

An uninformed person is at risk of mistakenly making a choice not reflective of his or her values or wishes.

Patients can elect to make their own medical decisions, or can delegate decision-making authority to another party.

If the patient is incapacitated, laws around the world designate different processes for obtaining informed consent, typically by having a person appointed by the patient or their next of kin make decisions for them.

The value of informed consent is closely related to the values of autonomy and truth telling.

A correlate to "informed consent" is the concept of informed refusal.

PATERNALISM

Many patients are not competent to make decisions for themselves; e.g., young children, individuals affected by certain psychiatric or neurological conditions, and those who are temporarily unconscious or comatose.

These patients require substitute decisionmakers, either the physician or another person.

Ethical issues arise in the determination of the appropriate substitute decision-maker and in the choice of criteria for decisions.

When medical paternalism prevailed, the physician was considered to be the appropriate decision-maker for incompetent patients.

Physicians might consult with family members about treatment options, but the final decisions were theirs to make.

Physicians have been gradually losing this authority in many countries as patients are given the opportunity to name their own substitute decisionmakers to act for them when they become incompetent.

In addition, some states specify the appropriate substitute decision-makers in descending order (e.g., husband or wife, adult children, brothers and sisters, etc.).

In such cases physicians make decisions for patients only when the designated substitute cannot be found, as in emergency situations.

The principles and procedures for informed consent are just as applicable to substitute decision-making as to patients making their own decisions.

Physicians have the same duty to provide all the information the substitute decision-makers need to make their decisions.

The principal criteria to be used for treatment decisions for an incompetent patient are his or her preferences, if these are known.

The preferences may be found in an advance directive or may have been communicated to the designated substitute decision-maker, the physician or other members of the healthcare team.

When an incompetent patient's preferences are not known, treatment decisions should be based on the patient's best interests, taking into account:

−The patient's diagnosis and prognosis.

−The patient's known values.

−Information received from those who are significant in the patient's life and who could help in determining his or her best interests.

−Aspects of the patient's culture and religion that would influence a treatment decision.

CONFIDENTIALITY

The physician's duty to maintain confidentiality means that a physician may not disclose any medical information revealed by a patient or discovered by a physician in connection with the treatment of a patient.

Legal protections prevent physicians from revealing their discussions with patients, even under oath in court.

A breach of confidentiality is a disclosure to a third party, without patient consent.

For example, in sexually transmitted disease in a patient who refuses to reveal the diagnosis to a spouse; and in the termination of a pregnancy in an underage patient, without the knowledge of the patient's parents.

Traditionally, medical ethics has viewed the duty of confidentiality as a relatively non-negotiable tenet of medical practice.

More recently, critics like Jacob Appel have argued for a more nuanced approach to the duty that acknowledges the need for flexibility in many cases.

Confidentiality is an important issue in primary care ethics, where physicians care for many patients from the same family and community, and where third parties often request information from the considerable medical database typically gathered in primary health care.

ABANDONMENT

There may be times, when a physician may no longer be able to provide care.

It may be that the patient is noncompliant, unreasonably demanding, threatening, or otherwise contributing to a breakdown in the physician-patient relationship.

It may be necessary to end the relationship simply due to relocation, retirement, or unanticipated termination by a managed care plan and/or employer.

Regardless of the situation, to avoid a claim of "patient abandonment", a physician must follow appropriate steps to terminate the physician-patient relationship.

Abandonment is defined as the termination of a professional relationship between physician and patient at an unreasonable time and without giving the patient the chance to find an equally qualified replacement.

Appropriate steps to terminate the physician-patient relationship typically include the following:

- Giving the patient notice, preferably by certified mail, return receipt requested.

- Providing the patient with a brief explanation for terminating the relationship (this should be a valid reason, for instance non-compliance, failure to keep appointments).

– Agreeing to continue to provide treatment and access to services for a reasonable period of time, such as 30 days, to allow a patient to secure care from another physician.

– Providing resources and/or recommendations to help a patient locate another physician of like specialty.

– Offering to transfer records to a newly-designated physician upon signed patient authorization to do so.

CONFLICTS OF INTEREST

Physicians should not allow a conflict of interest to influence medical judgment.

In some cases, conflicts are hard to avoid, and physicians have a responsibility to avoid entering such situations.

However, research has shown that conflicts of interests are very common among both academic physicians and physicians in practice.

Vendor Relationships

Studies show that physicians can be influenced by drug company inducements, including gifts and food.

Industry-sponsored Continuing Medical Education (CME) programs influence prescribing patterns.

Many patients surveyed in one study agreed that physician gifts from drug companies influence prescribing practices.

A growing movement among physicians is attempting to diminish the influence of pharmaceutical industry marketing upon medical practice, as evidenced by Stanford University's ban on drug company-sponsored lunches and gifts.

Other academic institutions have also banned pharmaceutical industry-sponsored gifts and food including the Johns Hopkins Medical Institutions, University of Michigan, University of Pennsylvania, and Yale University.

Referral

For example, physicians who receive income from referring patients for medical tests have been shown to refer more patients for medical tests.

This practice is proscribed by the American College of Physicians Ethics Manual.

Fee splitting and the payments of commissions to attract referrals of patients are considered unethical in most parts of the world.

Sexual Relationships

Sexual relationships between physicians and patients can create ethical conflicts, since sexual consent may conflict with the fiduciary responsibility of the physician.

Physicians who enter into sexual relationships with patients face the threats of deregistration and prosecution.

Sexual relationships between physicians and patients' relatives may also be prohibited in some jurisdictions, although this prohibition is highly controversial.

Treatment of Family Members

Physicians who do so must be vigilant not to create conflicts of interest or treat inappropriately.

CONTROL AND RESOLUTION

To ensure that appropriate ethical values are being applied within hospitals, effective hospital accreditation requires that ethical considerations are taken into account with respect to physician integrity, conflict of interest, research ethics and organ transplantation ethics.

Guidelines

There are various ethical guidelines, e.g., the Declaration of Helsinki is regarded as authoritative in human research ethics.

In the United Kingdom, General Medical Council provides clear overall modern guidance in the form of its 'Good Medical Practice' statement.

Other organisations, such as the Medical Protection Society and a number of university departments, are often consulted by British physicians regarding issues relating to ethics.

Ethics Committees

Often, simple communication is not enough to resolve a conflict, and a hospital ethics committee must convene to decide a complex matter.

These bodies are composed primarily of healthcare professionals, but may also include philosophers, lay people, and clergy - indeed, in many parts of the world their presence is considered mandatory in order to provide balance.

With respect to the expected composition of such bodies in the USA, Europe and Australia, the following applies.

U.S. recommendations suggest that Research and Ethical Boards (REBs) should have five or more members, including at least one scientist, one non-scientist, and one person not affiliated with the institution.

The REB should include people knowledgeable in the law and standards of practice and professional conduct.

The European Forum for Good Clinical Practice (EFGCP) suggests that REBs include two practicing physicians who share experience in biomedical research and are independent from the institution where the research is conducted; one lay person; one lawyer; and one paramedical professional, e.g., nurse or pharmacist.

The 1996 Australian Health Ethics Committee recommendations were entitled, "Membership Generally of Institutional Ethics Committees".

They suggest a chairperson be preferably someone not employed or otherwise connected with the institution.

Members should include a person with knowledge and experience in professional care, counselling or treatment of humans; a minister of religion or equivalent, e.g., Aboriginal elder; a layman; a laywoman; a lawyer and, in the case of a hospital-based ethics committee, a nurse.

CULTURAL ISSUES

Culture differences can create difficult medical ethics problems.

Some cultures have spiritual or magical theories about the origins of disease, and reconciling these beliefs with the tenets of Western medicine can be difficult.

Truth-Telling

Some cultures do not place a great emphasis on informing the patient of the diagnosis, especially when cancer is the diagnosis.

American culture rarely used truth-telling especially in medical cases, up until the 1970s.

In American medicine, the principle of informed consent now takes precedence over other ethical values, and patients are usually at least asked whether they want to know the diagnosis.

Online Business Practices

The delivery of diagnosis online leads patients to believe that physicians in some parts of the country are at the direct service of drug companies.

Finding diagnosis as convenient as what drug still has patent rights on it.

Physicians and drug companies are found to be competing for top ten search engine ranks to lower costs of selling these drugs with little to no patient involvement.

ETHICS IN BIO-INFORMATICS

In increasing frequency, medical researchers are researching activities in online environments such as discussion boards and bulletin boards, and there is concern that the requirements of informed consent and privacy are not as stringently applied as they should be, although some guidelines do exist.

One issue that has arisen, however, is the disclosure of information.

While researchers wish to quote from the original source in order to argue a point, this can have repercussions.

The quotations and other information about the site can be used to identify the site, and researchers have reported cases where members of the site, bloggers and others have used this information as 'clues' in a game in an attempt to identify the site.

Some researchers have employed various methods of "heavy disguise", including discussing a different condition from that under study, or even setting up bogus sites to ensure that the researched site is not discovered.

BEGINNING-OF-LIFE ISSUES

Many of the most prominent issues in medical ethics relate to the beginning of human life.

Each of these issues has been the subject of extensive analysis by medical associations, ethicists and government advisory bodies, and in many countries there are laws, regulations and policies dealing with them.

Contraception

There is increasing international recognition of a woman's right to control her fertility, including the prevention of unwanted pregnancies.

Physicians have to deal with difficult issues such as requests for contraceptives from minors and explaining the risks of different methods.

Assisted Reproduction

For couples (or individuals) who cannot conceive naturally there are various techniques of assisted reproduction, such as artificial insemination and IVF, widely available in major medical centres.

Surrogate or substitute gestation is another alternative.

None of these techniques is unproblematic, either in individual cases or for public policies.

Prenatal Genetic Screening

Genetic tests are now available for determining whether an embryo is affected by certain genetic abnormalities and whether it is male or female.

Depending on the findings, a decision can be made whether or not to proceed with pregnancy.

Physicians need to determine when to offer such tests and how to explain the results to patients.

Abortion

This has long been one of the most divisive issues in medical ethics, both for physicians and for public authorities.

Severely Compromised Neonates

Because of extreme prematurity or congenital abnormalities, some neonates have a very poor prognosis for survival.

Difficult decisions often have to be made whether to attempt to prolong their lives or allow them to die.

Research Issues

These include the production of new embryos or the use of "spare" embryos (those not wanted for reproductive purposes) to obtain stem cells for potential therapeutic applications, testing of new techniques for assisted reproduction, and experimentation on fetuses.

END-OF-LIFE ISSUES

End-of-life issues range from attempts to prolong the lives of dying patients through highly experimental technologies, such as the implantation of animal organs, to efforts to terminate life prematurely through euthanasia and medically assisted suicide.

In between these extremes lie numerous issues regarding the initiation or withdrawing of potentially life-extending treatments, the care of terminally ill patients and the advisability and use of advance directives.

Euthanasia

Euthanasia means knowingly and intentionally performing an act that is clearly intended to end another person's life and that includes the following elements:

− The subject is a competent, informed person with an incurable illness who has voluntarily asked for his or her life to be ended.

− The agent knows about the person's condition and desire to die, and commits the act with the primary intention of ending the life of that person.

− The act is undertaken with compassion and without personal gain.

Assistance in Suicide

Assistance in suicide means knowingly and intentionally providing a person with the knowledge or means or both required to commit suicide, including counselling about lethal doses of drugs, prescribing such lethal doses or supplying the drugs.

Euthanasia and assisted suicide are often regarded as morally equivalent, although there is a clear practical distinction, and in some jurisdictions a legal distinction, between them.

Euthanasia and assisted suicide, according to these definitions, are to be distinguished from the withholding or withdrawal of inappropriate, futile or unwanted medical treatment or the provision of compassionate palliative care, even when these practices shorten life.

Requests for euthanasia or assistance in suicide arise as a result of pain or suffering that is considered by the patient to be intolerable; they would rather die than continue to live in such circumstances.

Furthermore, many patients consider that they have a right to die if they so choose, and even a right to assistance in dying.

Physicians are regarded as the most appropriate instruments of death since they have the medical knowledge and access to the appropriate drugs for ensuring a quick and painless death.

Physicians are understandably reluctant to implement requests for euthanasia or assistance in suicide because these acts are illegal in most countries and are prohibited in most medical codes of ethics.

Euthanasia, that is the act of deliberately ending the life of a patient, even at the patient's own request or at the request of close relatives, is unethical.

This does not prevent the physician from respecting the desire of a patient to allow the natural process of death to follow its course in the terminal phase of sickness.

The rejection of euthanasia and assisted suicide does not mean that physicians can do nothing for the patient with a life-threatening illness at an advanced stage and for which curative measures are not appropriate.

Once physicians have made every effort to provide patients with information about the available treatments and their likelihood of success, they must respect the patients' decisions about the initiation or continuation of any treatment.

Futility

The concept of medical futility has been an important topic in discussions of medical ethics.

What should be done if there is no chance that a patient will survive but the family members insist on advanced care?

Previously, some articles defined futility as the patient having less than a one percent chance of surviving.

Advance directives include living wills and durable powers of attorney for health care.

In many cases, the "expressed wishes" of the patient are documented in these directives, and this provides a framework to guide family members and health care professionals in the decision making process when the patient is incapacitated.

"Substituted judgment" is the concept that a family member can give consent for treatment if the patient is unable (or unwilling) to give consent themselves.

The key question for the decision making surrogate is not, "What would you like to do?", but instead, "What do you think the patient would want in this situation?".

Courts have supported family's arbitrary definitions of futility to include simple biological survival, as in the Baby K case (in which the courts ordered a child born with only a brain stem instead of a complete brain to be kept on a ventilator based on the religious belief that all life must be preserved).

In some hospitals, medical futility is referred to as "non-beneficial care".

Baby Doe Law establishes state protection for a disabled child's right to life, ensuring that this right is protected even over the wishes of parents or guardians in cases where they want to withhold treatment.

CONTROVERSIES IN MEDICAL ETHICS

Double Effect

Double effect refers to two types of consequences that may be produced by a single action, and in medical ethics it is usually regarded as the combined effect of beneficence and non-maleficence.

A commonly cited example of this phenomenon is the use of morphine or other analgesic in the dying patient.

Such use of morphine can have the beneficial effect of easing the pain while simultaneously having the maleficent effect of shortening the life of the patient through suppression of the respiratory system.

Autonomy versus Beneficence/Non-Maleficence

Autonomy can come into conflict with beneficence when patients disagree with recommendations that healthcare professionals believe are in the patient's best interest.

When the patient's interests conflict with the patient's welfare, different societies settle the conflict in a wide range of manners.

In general, Western medicine defers to the wishes of a mentally competent patient to make his own decisions, even in cases where the medical team believes that he is not acting in his own best interests.

However, many other societies prioritize beneficence over autonomy, e.g., when a patient does not want a treatment because of religious or cultural views.

In the case of euthanasia, the patient, or relatives of a patient, may want to end the life of the patient.

Also, the patient may want an unnecessary treatment, as can be the case in hypochondria or with cosmetic surgery; here, the practitioner may be required to balance the desires of the patient for medically unnecessary potential risks against the patient's informed autonomy in the issue.

A physician may want to prefer autonomy because refusal to please the patient's will would harm the physician-patient relationship.

Individuals' capacity for informed decision making may come into question during resolution of conflicts between autonomy and beneficence.

The role of surrogate medical decision makers is an extension of the principle of autonomy.

On the other hand, autonomy and beneficence/non-maleficence may also overlap.

For example, a breach of patients' autonomy may cause decreased confidence for medical services in the population and subsequently less willingness to seek help, which in turn may cause inability to perform beneficence.

The principles of autonomy and beneficence/non-maleficence may also be expanded to include effects on the relatives of patients or even the medical practitioners, the overall population and economic issues when making medical decisions.

Criticisms of Orthodox Medical Ethics

It has been argued that mainstream medical ethics is biased by the assumption of a framework in which individuals are not simply free to contract with one another to provide whatever medical treatment is demanded, subject to the ability to pay.

Because a high proportion of medical care is typically provided via the welfare state, and because there are legal restrictions on what treatment may be provided and by whom, an automatic divergence may exist between the wishes of patients and the preferences of medical practitioners and other parties.

The idea that beneficence might in some cases have priority over autonomy has been questioned.

Violations of autonomy more often reflect the interests of the state or of the supplier group than those of the patient.

Routine regulatory professional bodies or the courts of law are valid social recourses.

MEDICAL RESEARCH ETHICS

Many prominent medical researchers in the 19th and 20th centuries conducted experiments on patients without their consent and with little if any concern for the patients' well-being.

Although there were some statements of research ethics dating from the early 20th century, they did not prevent physicians in Nazi Germany and elsewhere from performing research on subjects that clearly violated fundamental human rights.

Following World War Two, some of these physicians were tried and convicted by a special tribunal at Nuremberg, Germany.

The basis of the judgment is known as the Nuremberg Code, which has served as one of the foundational documents of modern research ethics.

Among the ten principles of this Code is the requirement of voluntary consent if a patient is to serve as a research subject.

A set of Principles for Those in Research and Experimentation was adopted as the Declaration of Helsinki (DoH) in 1964.

It was further revised in 1975, 1983, 1989, 1996, 2000 and 2008.

Despite the different scope, length and authorship of these documents, they agree to a very large extent on the basic principles of research ethics.

These principles have been incorporated in the laws and/or regulations of many countries and international organizations, including those that deal with the approval of drugs and medical devices.

Ethics Review Committee Approval

Paragraph 15 of the DoH stipulates that every proposal for medical research on human subjects must be reviewed and approved by an independent ethics committee before it can proceed.

In order to obtain approval, researchers must explain the purpose and methodology of the project; demonstrate how research subjects will be recruited, how their consent will be obtained and how their privacy will be protected; specify how the project is being funded; and disclose any potential conflicts of interest on the part of the researchers.

The ethics committee may approve the project as presented, require changes before it can start, or refuse approval altogether.

Many committees have a further role of monitoring projects that are underway to ensure that the researchers fulfil their obligations and they can if necessary stop a project because of serious unexpected adverse events.

The reason why ethics committee approval of a project is required is that neither researchers nor research subjects are always knowledgeable and objective enough to determine whether a project is scientifically and ethically appropriate.

Researchers need to demonstrate to an impartial expert committee that the project is worthwhile, that they are competent to conduct it, and that potential research subjects will be protected against harm to the greatest extent possible.

One unresolved issue regarding ethics committee review is whether a multi-centre project requires committee approval at each centre or whether approval by one committee is sufficient.

If the centres are in different countries, review and approval is generally required in each country.

Scientific Merit

Paragraph 12 of the DoH requires that medical research involving human subjects must be justifiable on scientific grounds.

This requirement is meant to eliminate projects that are unlikely to succeed, e.g., because they are methodologically inadequate, or that, even if successful, will likely produce trivial results.

If patients are being asked to participate in a research project, even where risk of harm is minimal, there should be an expectation that important scientific knowledge will be the result.

To ensure scientific merit, paragraph 12 requires that the project be based on a thorough knowledge of the literature on the topic and on previous laboratory and, where appropriate, animal research that gives good reason to expect that the proposed intervention will be efficacious in human beings.

All research on animals must conform to ethical guidelines that minimize the number of animals used and prevent unnecessary pain.

Paragraph 16 adds a further requirement - that only scientifically qualified persons should conduct research on human subjects.

The ethics review committee needs to be convinced that these conditions are fulfilled before it approves the project.

Social Value

One of the more controversial requirements of a medical research project is that it contribute to the wellbeing of society in general.

It used to be widely agreed that advances in scientific knowledge were valuable in themselves and needed no further justification.

However, as resources available for medical research are increasingly inadequate, social value has emerged as an important criterion for judging whether a project should be funded.

Paragraphs 17 and 21 of the DoH clearly favour the consideration of social value in the evaluation of research projects.

The importance of the project's objective, understood as both scientific and social importance, should outweigh the risks and burdens to research subjects.

Furthermore, the populations in which the research is carried out should benefit from the results of the research.

This is especially important in countries where there is potential for unfair treatment of research subjects who undergo the risks and discomfort of research while the drugs developed as a result of the research only benefit patients elsewhere.

The social worth of a research project is more difficult to determine than its scientific merit but that is not a good reason for ignoring it.

Researchers, and ethics review committees, must ensure that patients are not subjected to tests that are unlikely to serve any useful social purpose.

To do otherwise would waste valuable health resources and weaken the reputation of medical research as a major contributing factor to human health and well-being.

Risks and Benefits

Once the scientific merit and social worth of the project have been established, it is necessary for the researcher to demonstrate that the risks to the research subjects are not unreasonable or disproportionate to the expected benefits of the research, which may not even go to the research subjects.

A risk is the potential for an adverse outcome (harm) to occur.

It has two components:

- The likelihood of the occurrence of harm (from highly unlikely to very likely).

- The severity of the harm (from trivial to permanent severe disability or death).

A highly unlikely risk of a trivial harm would not be problematic for a good research project.

At the other end of the spectrum, a likely risk of a serious harm would be unacceptable unless the project provided the only hope of treatment for terminally ill research subjects.

In between these two extremes, paragraph 20 of the DoH requires researchers to adequately assess the risks and be sure that they can be managed.

If the risk is entirely unknown, then the researcher should not proceed with the project until some reliable data are available, e.g., from laboratory studies or experiments on animals.

Informed Consent

The first principle of the Nuremberg Code reads as follows: "The voluntary consent of the human subject is absolutely essential".

The explanatory paragraph attached to this principle requires, among other things, that the research subject "should have sufficient knowledge and comprehension of the elements of the subject matter involved as to enable him to make an understanding and enlightened decision".

The DoH goes into some detail about informed consent:

- Paragraph 24 specifies what the research subject needs to know in order to make an informed decision about participation.

- Paragraph 26 warns against pressuring individuals to participate in research, since in such circumstances the consent may not be entirely voluntary.

- Paragraphs 27 to 29 deal with research subjects who are unable to give consent (minor children, severely mentally handicapped individuals, unconscious patients); they can still serve as research subjects but only under restricted conditions.

The DoH, like other research ethics documents, recommends that informed consent be demonstrated by having the research subject sign a "consent form" (paragraph 24).

Many ethics review committees require the researcher to provide them with the consent form they intend to use for their project.

In some countries these forms have become so long and detailed that they no longer serve the purpose of informing the research subject about the project.

In any case, the process of obtaining informed consent does not begin and end with the form being signed but must involve a careful oral explanation of the project and all that participation in it will mean to the research subject.

Moreover, research subjects should be informed that they are free to withdraw their consent to participate at any time, even after the project has begun, without any sort of reprisal from the researchers or other physicians and without any compromise of their healthcare.

Confidentiality

As with patients in clinical care, research subjects have a right to privacy with regard to their personal health information.

Unlike clinical care, however, research requires the disclosure of personal health information to others, including the wider scientific community and sometimes the general public.

In order to protect privacy, researchers must ensure that they obtain the informed consent of research subjects to use their personal health information for research purposes.

This requires that the subjects are told in advance about the uses to which their information is going to be put.

As a general rule, the information should be de-identified and should be stored and transmitted securely.

Conflict of Roles

The physician's role in the physician-patient relationship is different from the researcher's role in the researcher-research subject relationship, even if the physician and the researcher are the same person.

Paragraph 31 of the DoH specifies that in such cases, the physician role must take precedence.

This means, among other things, that the physician must be prepared to recommend that the patient not take part in a research project if the patient seems to be doing well with the current treatment and the project requires that patients be randomized to different treatments and/or to a placebo.

Only if the physician, on solid scientific grounds, is truly uncertain whether the patient's current treatment is as suitable as a proposed new treatment, or even a placebo, should the physician ask the patient to take part in the research project.

Honest Reporting of Results

It should not be necessary to require that research results be reported accurately, but unfortunately there have been numerous recent accounts of dishonest practices in the publication of research results.

Problems include "plagiarism", data fabrication, duplicate publication and "gift" authorship.

Such practices may benefit the researcher, at least until they are discovered, but they can cause great harm to patients, who may be given incorrect treatments based on inaccurate or false research reports, and to other researchers, who may waste much time and resources trying to follow up the studies.

Whistle-Blowing

In order to prevent unethical research from occurring, or to expose it after the fact, anyone who has knowledge of such behaviour has an obligation to disclose this information to the appropriate authorities.

Unfortunately, such whistle-blowing is not always appreciated or even acted on, and whistle-blowers are sometimes punished or avoided for trying to expose wrong-doing.

This attitude seems to be changing, however, as both medical scientists and government regulators are seeing the need to detect and punish unethical research and are beginning to appreciate the role of whistle-blowers in achieving this goal.

Junior members of a research team, such as medical students, may find it especially difficult to act on suspicions of unethical research, since they may feel unqualified to judge the actions of senior researchers and will likely be subject to punishment if they speak out.

At the very least, however, they should refuse to participate in practices that they consider clearly unethical, e.g., lying to research subjects or fabricating data.

If they observe others engaging in such practices, they should take whatever steps they can to alert relevant authorities, either directly or anonymously.

Unresolved Issues

Not all aspects of research ethics enjoy general agreement.

As medical science continues to advance, in areas such as genetics, the neurosciences and organ and tissue transplantation, new questions arise regarding the ethical acceptability of techniques, procedures and treatments for which there are no ready-made answers.

Moreover, some older issues are still subjects of continuing ethical controversy, e.g., under what conditions should a placebo arm be included in a clinical trial and what continuing care should be provided to participants in medical research.

At a global level, the 10/90 gap in medical research (only 10% of global research funding is spent on health problems that affect 90% of the world's population) is clearly an unresolved ethical issue.

And when researchers do address problems in resource-poor areas of the world, they often encounter problems due to conflicts between their ethical outlook and that of the communities where they are working.

All these issues will require much further analysis and discussion before general agreement is achieved.

Despite all these potential problems, medical research is a valuable and rewarding activity for physicians and medical students as well as for the research subjects themselves.

Indeed, physicians and medical students should consider serving as research subjects so that they can appreciate the other side of the researcher-research subject relationship.

MEDICAL ERRORS

Medical errors are unentended, iatrogenic adverse effect resulting from medical management and leading to prolonged hospital stay, death or measurable disability at discharge.

Classification

Conceptual Errors

Unsound, contraindicated, or inapproriate medical approach.

Side Effects

Adverse effect of a correct medical approach:

− Preventable: e.g., failure of prophylaxis, failure to monitor or follow up treatment; lack of proper technical training.

− Non-preventable: acceptable side effects of correct medical approach, e.g., facial nerve injury in malignant parotid surgery.

Examples

Medical

− Medication errors, e.g., wrong drug, wrong dose, wrong patient, or wrong time or route of administration.

− Misdiagnosis, e.g., missing cancer colon in a patient with iron deficiency anaemia.

− Inappropriate treatment.

Surgical

– Technique-related.

– Postoperative bleeding.

– Retention of sponges/instruments.

– Wrong site/person/procedure surgery.

Pathogenesis

Problems may arise through:

Misidentification

– Mismatched transfusion.

– Wrong-site surgery.

– Wrong-person surgery.

– Wrong procedure.

Inexperience / Fatigue / Carelessness / Negligence

Inexperience of surgeons may result from:

– New technique or technology, e.g., laparoscopy, which requires training.

– Incompetence of the surgeon, leading to higher rate of conceptual errors).

<u>System Failure</u>

The errors generated by an incompetent surgeon must be distinguished from those resulting from system failure.

Traditional medical culture considers errors as an individual problem and blames the responsible physician.

A system approach, as applied in industry, has shown that medical errors are often the result of system failure.

The individual components of patient care constitute a system (interdependent items or functions which constitute a whole).

How to Improve Patient Safety?

−Avoid clerical errors by checking and double-checking names, drugs and their doses, marking operation sites.

−Do not perform procedures you are not experienced with, ask for a senior to supervise or assist you.

−Use standard procedures to improve patient safety, e.g., appropriate use of prophylaxis to prevent thrombo-embolism in patients at risk, appropriate use of antibiotic prophylaxis to prevent postoperative infection.

−Use a system approach by defining the various components of patient care and the errors that can possibly occur as each component is implemented, e.g., marking the site of an operation, checking lab results, quality assurance protocols for labs; instrument maintenance.

Relevance to Medical Ethics

Conceptual Errors

Violate the ethical principles of:

– Beneficience

– Non-maleficience

– Truth telling

Non-Conceptual but Preventable Side Effects

Raise the issues of:

– Negligence (associated substandard care).

– Incompetence (violates beneficience through not referring the patient to more competent physician).

Errors due to System Failure

Complications related to, e.g.:

– Inaccurate lab results

– Poor quality instruments/equipment

– Laisser-aller attitude of administration (non-observance of rules).

MEDICAL ETHICS EDUCATION

A background in ethics has long been recognized as an important credential for medical professionals.

Over the past years, training in ethics has been incorporated into the medical curriculum, albeit with little regulation.

Since recent advancements in medical care are associated with complex ethical issues, it is important that medical students, residents, and practicing physicians learn and understand ethics within a framework that is well-founded, rigorous, and longitudinally based.

While it may be safe to assume that most people who enter the profession will have their own moral code, physicians still need to keep up with the increasingly complex ethical dilemmas of modern medicine.

A unified framework of ethics education ensures a measurable and accountable basis for the complex and far-reaching ethical issues present in the medical field.

Medical educators in Canada, the UK and Australia have reached consensus on aspects of ethics education in their respective countries including core values, curriculum, and teaching methods.

The United States needs to reach consensus and then take the next step of national implementation.

In 2006 the American Medical Association (AMA) launched Innovative Strategies for Transforming the Education of Physicians (ISTEP).

As a first step, medical educators in the United States may want to evaluate where the instillation of ethical values seems to have failed.

Perhaps a review of reasons for revocation of medical licenses or expulsion from medical schools and residency programs would reveal areas in most urgent need of attention.

Additionally, reviewing complaints brought against physicians by patients, colleagues, and others may demonstrate shortcomings in ethical instruction.

A review by a committee of medical educators of subject material currently being taught at the medical student and resident level could produce a consensus statement as to which specific topics in ethics could be taught.

Finally, comparing these topics to those already being addressed overseas could produce a core ethics curriculum which could be implemented into medical student and residency training, with a focus on small group and clinical case-based discussions.

This could then be followed by rigorous evaluation of teaching methods and outcomes, with a goal of continuous process improvement.

This may assure that certain specific fundamental ethical principles have been addressed during medical training, and that failures in ethical behavior among practicing physicians are not due to shortcomings in medical education.

FUTURE OF MEDICAL ETHICS

The future of medical ethics will depend in large part on the future of medicine.

The future will not necessarily be better than the present, given widespread political and economic instability, environmental degradation, the continuing spread of epidemics.

Given the inherent unpredictability of the future, medical ethics needs to be flexible and open to change and adjustment, as indeed it has been for some time now.

Whatever changes in medicine occur as a result of scientific developments and social, political and economic factors, there will always be sick people needing cure if possible and care always.

Physicians have traditionally provided these services along with others such as health promotion, disease prevention and health system management.

Although the balance among these activities may change in the future, physicians will likely continue to play an important role in all of them.

Since each activity involves many ethical challenges, physicians will need to keep informed about developments in medical ethics just as they do in other aspects of medicine.

REFERENCES

– Abrams N, Buckner M. Medical Ethics. Cambridge: MIT Press; 1983.

– Beauchamp T, Childress J. Principles of Biomedical Ethics. New York: Oxford University Press; 2001.

– Bekelman J, Li Y, Gross C. Scope and impact of financial conflicts of interest in biomedical research: a systematic review. JAMA. 2003; 289: 454-65.

– Blake R, Early E. Patients' attitudes about gifts to physicians from pharmaceutical companies. J Am Board Fam Pract. 1995; 8: 457-64.

– Brody B. Life and Death Decision Making. New York: Oxford University Press; 1988.

– Brody H. Ethical Decisions in Medicine. Boston: Little, Brown & Com; 1981.

– Bruckman A. Studying the amateur artist: A perspective on disguising data collected in human subjects' research on the Internet. Ethics and Information Technology. 2002; 4: 217-31.

– Culver C, Gert B. Philosophy in Medicine. New York: Oxford University Press; 1982.

– Dubois J, Burkemper J. Ethics education in U.S. medical schools: A study of syllabi. Acad Med. 2002; 77: 432-7.

– Eckles R, Meslin E, Gaffney M, Helft P. Medical Ethics Education: Where Are We? Where Should We Be? A Review. Acad Med. 2005; 80: 1143-52.

– Elahi M. Medical Ethics - A Practical guide to patient care related ethics, conventions and laws. MTRO Publishing, Pakistan, 2011.

– Elcin M, Odabasi O, Gokler B, Sayek I, Akova M, Kiper N. Developing and evaluating professionalism. Med Teach. 2006; 28: 36-9.

– Epstein S. Inclusion: The Politics of Difference in Medical Research. University of Chicago Press; 2009.

– Eysenbach G, Till J. Ethical issues in qualitative research on internet communities. BMJ. 2001; 323: 1103-5.

– Gartrell N, Milliken N, Goodson W, Thiemann S, Lo B. Physician-patient sexual contact. Prevalence and problems. West J Med. 1992; 157: 139-43.

– General Assembly of the World Medical Association. World Medical Association Declaration of Helsinki: ethical principles for medical research involving human subjects. J Am Coll Dent. 2014; 81: 14-8.

– Gillon R. Principles of Health Care Ethics. Chichester: John Wiley & Sons; 1994.

– Gillon R. Defending the four principles approach as a good basis for good medical practice and therefore for good medical ethics. J Med Ethics. 2015; 41: 111-6.

– Giordano J, Schatman M. A crisis in chronic pain care - An ethical analysis. Part two: Proposed structure and function of an ethics of pain medicine. Pain Physician. 2008; 11: 589-95.

– Güldal D, Semin S. The influences of drug companies' advertising programs on physicians. Int J Health Serv. 2000; 30: 585-95.

– Howe E. How to retain the trust of patients and families when we will not provide the treatment they want. J Clin Ethics. 2015; 26: 89-99.

– Jordan M. Ethics manual. Fourth edition. American College of Physicians. Ann Intern Med. 1998; 128: 576-94.

– Kimmelman J, Weijer C, Meslin E. Helsinki discords: FDA, ethics, and international drug trials. The Lancet. 2009; 373: 13-4.

– Lakhan S, Hamlat E, McNamee T, Laird C. Time for a unified approach to medical ethics. Philos Ethics Humanit Med. 2009; 4: 13-5.

– Mappes T, Zembaty J. Biomedical Ethics. New York: McGraw Hill; 1991.

– Masic I, Hodzic A, Mulic S. Ethics in medical research and publication. Int J Prev Med. 2014; 5: 1073-82.

– Monagle J, Thomasma D. Medical Ethics. Rockville: Aspen Pub; 1988.

– Pellegrino E. Professionalism, profession and the virtues of the good physician. Mt Sinai J Med. 2002; 69: 378-84.

– Pellegrino E, Thomasma D. For the Patient's Good. New York: Oxford University Press; 1988.

– Pollard B. Autonomy and paternalism in medicine. The Medical journal of Australia. 1993; 159: 797-802.

– Randall F. Ethical issues in cancer pain management. In: Sykes N, Bennett MI, Yuan C-S. Clinical pain management: Cancer pain. Second edition. London: Hodder Arnold; 2008.

– Ross J, Lackner J, Lurie P, Gross C, Wolfe S, Krumholz H. Pharmaceutical company payments to physicians: early experiences with disclosure laws in Vermont and Minnesota. JAMA. 2007; 297: 1216-23.

– Ryan C. Ethical issues, part 2: ethics, psychiatry, and end-of-life issues. Psychiatr Times. 2010; 27: 26-7.

– Sherwin S. No Longer Patient: Feminist Ethics and Health Care. Philadelphia: Temple University Press; 1992.

– Swedlow A, Johnson G, Smithline N, Milstein A. Increased costs and rates of use in the California workers' compensation system as a result of self-referral by physicians. N Engl J Med. 1992; 327: 1502-6.

– Tassano F. The Power of Life or Death: Medical Coercion and the Euthanasia Debate. Oxford: Oxford Forum; 1999.

– Tauber A. Confessions of a Medicine Man. Cambridge: MIT Press; 1999.

– Tauber A. Patient Autonomy and the Ethics of Responsibility. Cambridge: MIT Press; 2005.

– Turkle S. Constructions and Reconstructions of Self in Virtual Reality. Mind, Culture, and Activity 1994; 1: 158-67.

– Turkle S. Multiple subjectivity and virtual community at the end of the Freudian century. Sociological Inquiry. 1997; 67: 72-84.

– UNESCO. Universal Declaration on Bioethics and Human Rights. Adopted by the UNESCO General Conference, Paris, 2005.

– Veatch R. A Theory of Medical Ethics. New York: Basic Books; 1988.

– Veatch R. Medical Ethics. Boston: Jones & Bartlett; 1989.

– Wallace M, Siersema P. Ethics in publication. Endoscopy. 2015; 47: 575-8.

– Walter J, Eran P. The Story of Bioethics: From seminal works to contemporary explorations. Georgetown University Press; 2003.

www.ingramcontent.com/pod-product-compliance
Lightning Source LLC
Chambersburg PA
CBHW070847180526
45168CB00002B/979